I0096649

HEALTH BEYOND LIP SERVICE

A 25-Day Journey to Faith-Based Wellness

LA'WANA HARRIS

Library of Congress Control Number: 2022921364

Copyright © 2022 La'Wana Harris.

All rights reserved. This book or any portion thereof may not be reproduced or used in any manner whatsoever without the express written permission of the publisher except for the use of brief quotations in a book review.

CONTENTS

INTRODUCTION

Welcome, my friends; I'm excited that you're joining me on this journey towards a healthier mind, body, and spirit. As you probably know, health is a struggle for many of us. Despite knowing some of the actions we must take to nourish our bodies and protect our mental health, many of us can't help but allow ourselves to drop to the bottom of our own list of priorities, because of our chaotic lifestyles and busy routines. This has to change and is why I prepared this devotional.

Obesity, for example, is a massive problem in America, and the numbers are alarming. The U.S. is ranked 12th among the countries with the highest percentage of obese people, and data from the CDC – Central for Disease Control – tell us that around 36,9% of American adults are overweight. Not to mention the problem of child obesity, which keeps increasing every year.

Also, the majority of people living with obesity are Black Americans. The CDC still says almost 50% of non-Hispanic black adults in the United States are obese. That's essentially **half of the black American population**! Even then, the same data suggests that non-Hispanic black women also have a higher obesity rate when compared to non-Hispanic black men.

But what does this matter?

Obesity is a risk factor for so many other complications, and it is extremely worrying that we're putting ourselves at risk of developing life-threatening illnesses. Something needs to change, and the best place to find answers, for believers, is our faith. Don't be mistaken; a healthy body is a sacred territory. Some Christians are often told to focus on the spiritual, which ends up minimizing the role of the physical. But the truth is both spirit and body matter when glorifying God?

Everything in our lives must reveal our connection with God, including the things we eat and drink. With each decision, each meal, and each practice, we're honoring Him. Just like one should be disciplined in reading the Bible and praying, we should also ensure that our bodies are healthy. However, we must be mindful that God isn't calling us all to have "perfect" health or "perfect" bodies, but instead, to cherish the breathing and living bodies we were given.

Our bodies are the ultimate gift from God, which is why we should make the conscious decision to not "trash" or destroy them. We should do our best to steward this gift. But how? Some of us have so many things to do every single day, and it can be an extremely difficult to change our health and habits. "**Health Beyond Lip Service**" was written as a devotional for the busy Christian women who can't afford to spend hours at the gym.

Following God's calling to honor Him by cherishing the gift of our bodies, I've prepared a **25-Days devotional journey**, which includes prayers, devotions, and tips that can be implemented and followed by even the busiest readers. I invite you to open your mind to this opportunity and walk with me while I show you that a faith-based approach to a healthier body—backed by research—is the best alternative there is.

Although so many programs designed to help Black women have had mixed results, studies have shown that because religion is such a prominent aspect of Black culture, it should be included as a crucial aspect of any weight loss/wellness strategy.

In a 12-week faith-based weight loss intervention conducted at the John H. Stroger, Jr. Hospital of Cook County in Chicago, titled Faith on the Move, obese black women had better overall results. The intervention was delivered in a small group format and met twice weekly for 12 weeks. Time was spent instructing and encouraging the use of tools, such as daily self-monitoring of food intake and physical activity, reinforcement, modeling, stimulus control, and social support, during the intervention. Additionally, a scripture was incorporated each week into the content of the intervention.

There is growing evidence that religious involvement has the ability to positively influence healthy behavior in black populations, and spiritual/religious beliefs have been demonstrated to play a significant role in how blacks—particularly black females—structure their lives.

Why is that?

Because ultimately, a Christian's life is meant to honor and glorify God. Every single day, when we wake up, choose what we're going to eat, how we're going to move our bodies, and how we're going to take care of ourselves, it must be to His honor. As Christians, the Holy Spirit dwells in our bodies, and when we nourish our bodies and take care of ourselves, we're creating a comfortable space for the Spirit to work within us.

Our bodies are God's temple, and it's our duty to take care of them.

Health Beyond Lip Service was written so that you can take care of the only body you'll ever have. Think about it! We place value on things that are scarce, but your body is the one and only temple you'll ever have. It cannot be replaced, so it must be treated well and with kindness. It must be a priority, as it is a way of honoring God.

Welcome, and I hope you find great value in this journey!

DAY 01

"Or do you not know that your body is a temple of the Holy Spirit within you, whom you have from God? You are not your own, for you were bought with a price. So glorify God in your body."

1 Corinthians 6:19,20 ESV

I'm no stranger to how overwhelming life can be. Most of us are almost drowning in responsibilities, and being able to handle everything while still looking after ourselves can quickly become a challenge. Most people are familiar with this feeling: waking up in the morning, and all you can think about is the long list of things you must take care of.

That's why we set priorities. Each of the decisions we make on a daily basis follows a priority order which we have previously set for ourselves, even if not intentionally. This verse is a reminder that we must be intentional in taking care of our bodies, as they are the temple of God.

When we have no regard for our health, we dishonor the Holy Spirit, and we're purposely leading ourselves to poor health. If we intend to use our body as a tool to glorify Him, then we must cherish it as a priority.

FAITH-BASED APPROACH: When you wake up every morning, make the conscious decision to be mindful of the things you're eating and drinking. Mindful Eating is a powerful tool, and it adds only a couple minutes to your meal time.

Instead of being distracted by your smartphone or TV while eating, focus on the food that's in front of you. Take this moment as an opportunity to honor God. Breathe calmly, **eat slowly, and appreciate the meal**. This will allow you to listen to your hunger cues instead of "devouring" a plate of food.

NOTES

_____

_____

_____

_____

_____

_____

_____

_____

_____

_____

_____

_____

_____

_____

_____

_____

DAY 02

*"But he answered, "It is written, Man shall not live by bread
alone, but by every word that comes from the mouth of God"."*
Matthew 4:4 ESV

Many Christians make the mistake of believing the body isn't as important as the Spirit. While most of us set aside some time to pray and honor God, we end up letting ourselves go. This verse highlights the importance of finding a proper balance between the physical, mental, and spiritual, which is why it is so valuable.

We need to eat and drink well to keep our bodies strong so that we are able to use them to honor God. We also need to be mentally strong and resilient, and that is only possible through the word of God, as He is the guide to our spiritual life. Whenever you feel tempted to break a promise made to yourself, you must be reminded that Jesus was never easily convinced by what seemed like tempting offers.

Both mental and physical strength can be achieved with the guidance of God, which is why one must not only feed their minds with God's words but also feed their bodies with the best food.

FAITH-BASED APPROACH: Nature is a powerful thing. Our ancestors, for example, were able to live by collecting the ingredients and foods directly from God's given earth. With time, this has changed, and we've become so addicted to eating products instead of food.

The best food for your body isn't necessarily a product made by thousands of machines but the ingredients provided by the earth. Try to **reduce the amount of processed and ultra-processed foods** in your pantry. Start by challenging yourself to cook at least one meal a day with only natural ingredients. Focus on peeling ingredients rather than opening packages.

NOTES

_____

_____

_____

_____

_____

_____

_____

_____

_____

_____

_____

_____

_____

_____

_____

_____

_____

_____

_____

DAY 03

*"So, whether you eat or drink, or whatever
you do, do all to the glory of God."*
1 Corinthians 10:31 ESV

We all must eat to survive. Many of us have a minimum of three meals a day, so it's normal that, at some point, we start to eat mindlessly, without paying much attention to what we're eating. We enter pilot mode, and forget about the importance of our meals and the things we are choosing to put in our bodies.

Eating well means glorifying God, but it requires a certain amount of control. He doesn't want us to destroy our bodies by consuming vast amounts of alcohol or drugs, and He doesn't want us to get carried away in our eating habits. You shouldn't eat something just because it's expensive or just because you want to "fit in."

The goal of eating is to honor God, and this verse explicitly calls for a mindful decision when choosing the things that we're eating so that we can avoid choosing to consume foods and drinks that won't do our bodies good.

FAITH-BASED APPROACH: For busy women, one of the biggest challenges is keeping track of what they are eating. So many of us are trying to do multiple things at once, making sure our kids are eating well and that everything is in order. As a result, we end up eating "whatever is there" without paying much attention.

In order to be more mindful about the things you're eating, **planning the meal** ahead of time can be of great help. Choose a day of the week when you're "less busy" and write down the meals for the week. This way, you won't have to struggle thinking and deciding what you're going to eat in the middle of a chaotic and busy day.

NOTES

_____

_____

_____

_____

_____

_____

_____

_____

_____

_____

_____

_____

_____

_____

_____

_____

DAY 04

*"It is not good to eat much honey, nor is it
glorious to seek one's own glory."*
Proverbs 25:27 ESV

This verse is all about modesty. The world is full of temptations, and as humans, we might feel overly attached to certain things to the point where we want to indulge in them. However, it's important to be mindful of such behaviors since scriptures are very explicit about overindulging.

Verse 16 of this very same chapter provides additional guidance, "If you have found honey, eat only enough for you, lest you have your fill of it and vomit it." Overeating is a massive problem, and when trying to eat healthier or lose weight in order to take care of our bodies, it's one of the first habits that we might want to change.

Especially because overeating isn't only harmful to the body but also to the mind. You shouldn't become obsessed with your meals, because they should only be an opportunity to nourish your body and not serve as an "escape mechanism."

FAITH-BASED APPROACH: Luckily, healthier foods can often be eaten in larger quantities when compared to what are considered to be fast foods. Thus, it shouldn't be difficult to control the portions of a healthier meal. However, there are still a couple of things one can do to ensure they're not overindulging.

It shouldn't take much time out of your day. You can start by **reducing the size of your plate**. Our brains don't appreciate the image of "emptiness," which means that the bigger the plate, the more food you'll serve. The opposite is also true. Alternatively, you can also ensure at least **half of your plate contains a low-calorie option**, such as a nutrient-dense salad.

NOTES

_____

_____

_____

_____

_____

_____

_____

_____

_____

_____

_____

_____

_____

_____

_____

_____

DAY 05

"And God said, "Behold, I have given you every plant yielding seed that is on the face of all the earth, and every tree with seed in its fruit. You shall have them for food."
Genesis 1:29 ESV

When God created Adam and Eve, all of the things that they needed to survive and thrive were already provided. He didn't create proper food and water later; but instead, they could already find everything they needed on earth. It works the same for us.

The earth provides us with the best quality food there is, including fruits, seeds, plants, and vegetables, which are essential to nourish our bodies. Thus, our diets should reflect God's desire as much as possible in order to maintain our health. God was extremely intentional in providing everything we needed for sustenance and wellbeing, so we should make use of it.

With this in mind, we can follow the Lord's provision for a healthier body, which is making the best use of the herbs, fruits, spices, fruits, and vegetables that are available in their most organic form.

FAITH-BASED APPROACH: Throughout the years, food was slowly modified for mass production. Instead of being consumed immediately, products now had to "last" for months before they could reach the supermarket's shelf. This was only possible with the addition of countless chemicals.

I'm aware that organic options are sometimes more expensive, and they can also be harder to find. However, it's worth making an effort to not only ensure that your diet is rich in spices, fruits, vegetables, and herbs but that they are also **organic** when possible. Organic foods reduce the risk of diseases, and they are overall more nutritious, containing more Vitamin C, Iron, Magnesium, and Phosphorus.

NOTES

_____

_____

_____

_____

_____

_____

_____

_____

_____

_____

_____

_____

_____

_____

_____

_____

DAY 06

"And the Lord spoke to Moses and Aaron, saying to them, ²"
Speak to the people of Israel, saying, These are the living things
that you may eat among all the animals that are on the earth.
³Whatever parts the hoof and is cloven-footed and chews the
cud, among the animals, you may eat."
Leviticus 11:1-3 ESV

God knows everything, and He, even more than ourselves, knows what's best for us and our bodies, which is why He made sure to describe in detail the things we could and couldn't eat, as this verse highlights. God knows the impact certain things will have on our bodies, and He wishes us no harm, which is why we should follow his guidance.

God categorized animals into two different types: clean and unclean, and He was very descriptive of the things he expected us to eat. The most important takeaway is that, just like God was selective about the things He expects us to eat, we must also be selective about the things we consume.

When we eat mindlessly and carelessly select our foods, God's guidance on what we should eat is disregarded. Thus, it's important that, when trying to live a healthier lifestyle, we are equally selective about the things we choose to buy and consume.

FAITH-BASED APPROACH: In moments of distress, one of the things we might feel tempted to do is run to our pantry and eat the most caloric fast food we can find. "Comfort foods" are often able to provide us with the immediate relief that we're so desperately craving.

These moments are often in the way of our attempts to become more selective about the things we're eating, as you're temporarily blinded by the overwhelming emotion you are feeling. A simple way to prevent this from becoming a habit is to **reduce the amount of junk food available in your pantry.** If you don't have it, chances are you won't buy it and will instead shift your attention to other alternatives to soothe your heart, like prayers.

NOTES

_____

_____

_____

_____

_____

_____

_____

_____

_____

_____

_____

_____

_____

_____

_____

_____

_____

DAY 07

"But Daniel resolved that he would not defile himself with the king's food, or with the wine that he drank. Therefore, he asked the chief of the eunuchs to allow him not to defile himself."
Daniel 1:8 ESV

This verse is all about simplicity, which is something that we're lacking in our diets. Be mindful, however, not to confuse simplicity with convenience. The most convenient meal for a lot of families is to simply order out or buy fast food, and that might not be ideal if you're trying to eat healthily.

Instead, simplicity is all about not overthinking your meals and ingredients and choosing to follow a simple and yet effective diet with natural foods. Daniel and his three friends are the best examples of this. Instead of having a lavish diet, they instead followed a simple diet plan which contained mostly vegetables and water.

Chapter fifteen of the same chapter says: *"At the end of ten days it was seen that they were better in appearance and fatter in flesh than all the youths who ate the king's food."* This essentially means that simple meals are the best option to provide happiness and health, not that healthy eating habits are a "luxury."

FAITH-BASED APPROACH: Not confusing simplicity with convenience is a challenge, but even in the busiest schedules, there are some things you can do in order to have fresh fruits and vegetables at your disposal. Having your fridge packed with healthy foods will reduce the frequency in which you consume high-calorie fast food.

The best approach here is to plan your meals ahead of time. On day 3, we saw the importance of planning your meals. You can also cook ahead of time. This will not only improve the quality of your diet but save you lots of time! You can even prepare salads in advance! **Choose a day of the week when you're less busy to be your official "cooking day,"** and mass prepare meals for as many days as you want. You can store the ones you'll eat in the next couple of days in the fridge and the remaining ones in the freezer.

NOTES

DAY 08

"You shall serve the Lord your God, and he will bless your bread and your water, and I will take sickness away from among you."
Exodus 23:25 ESV

This passage is all about reminding ourselves that God is our source of health, happiness, and wellness. It's about reminding ourselves that it is God who blesses our foods and drinks, which are then able to fortify and strengthen our bodies. It's a great passage to remind ourselves that we can always seek Him, as he has promised to remove sickness and provide health.

For this day, I want to remind us about the importance of praying or thanking Him for our meals. When Jesus miraculously fed countless people with only a few loaves and fish, he gave thanks. He then, again, fed 5,000 people with only five loaves of bread and two fish. At the Last Supper, yet again, Jesus gave thanks. His apostles, such as Paul, continued the practice of praying or giving thanks before eating.

When we are reminded to thank Him for providing us with food, we're acknowledging that our meals came from Him, and we recognize Him as the source of all that we have. Praying before meals is a habit that reminds us of this truth and, therefore, shouldn't be forgotten.

FAITH-BASED APPROACH: On day 01, we briefly mentioned the power of Mindful Eating. This tool is all about being aware of what you're doing, what you're thinking, and what you're eating. It's so easy to reach the dinner table "starving" and devour everything that's in front of us. Instead, I challenge you to reconsider this behavior.

Before jumping on your meal, **take a brief second to say thanks and give a prayer**. This simple and yet powerful habit is often forgotten, but it's an opportunity to honor God and acknowledge His efforts of providing for us. Ultimately, it raises awareness about our meals, allowing us to look at them in a healthier way instead of mindlessly eating without much thought. Thus, don't forget to be thankful to Him.

NOTES

DAY 09

"Beloved, I pray that all may go well with you and that you
may be in good health, as it goes well with your soul."
3 John 1:2 ESV

Our health and our wellbeing go hand in hand. When we're healthy, both physically and mentally, we're able to be happier, more optimistic, and more willing. On the other hand, when we're unhealthy, we often become depressed, sad, and hopeless. This verse is all about the connection between our health and wellness and why it is so important to cater to our health.

Throughout the day, we're often way too busy handling everything in our lives, that we sometimes end up not eating well. We drink too much coffee, and we mostly snack instead of properly sitting down to have a meal. It's not our fault, as we might be so overwhelmed by the number of things we need to do and the piling number of responsibilities waiting for us.

For many of us, the only "moment of peace" is at night, after the kids are finally sleeping and we are left alone for a couple of hours before we finally surrender to our comfortable bed. And that's when the habit of noshing at night can quickly make us gain weight.

FAITH-BASED APPROACH: Regardless of what type of diet one decides to follow, most approaches make it clear that eating big amounts of food at night before bed is not the best idea. However, it's not only about how much you eat but also about what you're eating when you're snacking at night.

After dinner, you can make an effort to think of the kitchen as "officially closed until the morning." Brushing your teeth also helps since it signals your body that you're done eating for the day. As an alternative, you can **leave a little plate of fruit by your bedside** in case you become hungry. Avoiding overeating at night will prevent trouble with digestion and bloating and help with weight management.

NOTES

DAY 10

"And rising very early in the morning, while it was still dark, he departed and went out to a desolate place, and there he prayed."
Mark 1:35 ESV

The decision to become healthier and take care of our bodies is a daily challenge that begins from the moment we wake up to the moment we go to bed. This passage is all about the importance of the morning, and that's precisely what we must be reminded of. What we do during the day will deeply affect our decisions for the remainder of the day.

This is why it is crucial to not only have healthy habits in the morning but to make efforts to ensure that making healthier decisions will be as easy as possible. When it comes to our diets, it all starts with breakfast. Mothers are often running around in the morning trying to make sure all kids are fed and ready for school, and sometimes skip breakfast themselves.

However, a proper breakfast is the ideal kick starter for your metabolism, which will ensure that you're burning enough calories for the rest of the day. A good quality breakfast will also provide you with all the energy and fuel you need. Along with your breakfast, taking a few minutes to say a prayer, just as suggested on Day 08. It is also extremely important. Never forget to give thanks!

FAITH-BASED APPROACH: Without the proper fuel provided by a good breakfast, there's a higher chance that you'll overeat later on in the day. Thus, even if you're in a rush, **try to make sure you're eating something easy and healthy**, such as fruits, yogurt, homemade smoothies, and cereal bars.

People who skip breakfast tend to gain more weight than those who don't, so it's important that you set eating well in the morning as a priority, even if you have to wake up a little earlier.

NOTES

DAY 11

*"And Jesus increased in wisdom and in stature
and in favor with God and man."*
Luke 2:52 ESV

Since one cannot fully exist without the other, I firmly believe that the true definition of health involves a well-balanced middle ground between physical and mental health. This passage, in particular, is a great reminder of this, as we are able to learn that Jesus was not only physically well, He was also confident and had great wisdom.

Mental wellness is also discussed in Daniel 2:20, where it reads, *"And in every matter of wisdom and understanding about which the king inquired of them, he found them ten times better than all the magicians and enchanters that were in all his kingdom."* The Hebrew brothers were healthy in every sense of the term. They were strong physically, mentally, and spiritually.

This is achievable with the help of a proper diet, an exercise routine, and constant communication with God, as He is the only one who can strengthen our spirits. Thus, it is of crucial importance that we make efforts to spiritually connect with God every day.

FAITH-BASED APPROACH: I've mentioned the importance of mindful eating on a couple of occasions by now, but you might be surprised to know that Mindful Eating is a subject of a broader term called **Mindfulness.** When talking about having a proper balance between body, spirit, and mind, mindfulness is a great opportunity.

It's hard to slow down and pay attention to what's happening around us, so doing some mindfulness exercises can help. One of them is a simple walk. Mindfulness challenges people to walk while paying attention to the smells, the feeling of their feet touching the ground, and the noise from the streets with a higher focus than before. **Going on Mindfulness walks** is not only beneficial to get your body moving, it is also great for improving sleep, attention and reducing burnout.

NOTES

_____

_____

_____

_____

_____

_____

_____

_____

_____

_____

_____

_____

_____

_____

_____

_____

_____

DAY 12

"I appeal to you therefore, brothers, by the mercies of God,
to present your bodies as a living sacrifice, holy and acceptable
to God, which is your spiritual worship."
Romans 12:1 ESV

Romans 12:1 is yet another verse that makes me reflect on the importance of taking care of my body. It is a great reminder that my health and wellness should be a priority, even in the middle of a chaotic and busy lifestyle. Our bodies ought to be living sacrifices that are holy and acceptable to God, so it's crucial that we are intentional and careful.

Just like you, I've had moments when becoming more active seemed like such a struggle. I had no time, no energy, and no will to spend hours at the gym. It took me a while to realize that I really didn't need to and that people have different realities. I was then willing to find solutions that worked for me and allowed me to take care of my body with the resources that I had available.

I decided that I didn't really need to "workout" and that being active simply meant moving my body more frequently. I could do this while also handling my everyday responsibilities.

FAITH-BASED APPROACH: Simple decisions such as going on daily walks, even if they are short, can already make a huge difference. **The most important thing is not to stay still and sit around for longer periods of time.** What might work for you is finding ways to move while going about your day. Here are a few suggestions:

- Make sure that you're taking the stairs instead of the elevator;
- Parking a couple stops before or after your destination and walking the rest of the way;
- Do more things yourself. These days we can hire someone to blow-dry our hair, do our nails, etc. But these activities can be fun while making your move more often.

NOTES

_____

_____

_____

_____

_____

_____

_____

_____

_____

_____

_____

_____

_____

_____

_____

_____

_____

_____

DAY 13

*"I have the right to do anything," you say—but not
everything is beneficial. "I have the right to do anything"
—but I will not be mastered by anything."*
1 Corinthians 6:12 ESV

This is a powerful verse that speaks to those who have ever felt like food was in control of their lives. I sure can relate to this feeling, and I'm certain many women feel the same: when we can't control our cravings, and we are blinded by the momentary "sense of happiness" that food can provide, but that fails to fulfill our souls the way we actually crave the most.

While thinking about following a better diet, eating well, and changing habits, I hope we all understand that nothing is completely off-limits but that we shouldn't be controlled by food. It's the other way around. It's up to us to put reasonable and healthy limits on the foods we eat.

In the same way that it is not good to go hours without eating, as our bodies will weaken and become susceptible to sicknesses, it is also not good to eat an entire chocolate cake or massive amounts of French fries. YOU have the right to choose what you're going to eat and in what quantity.

FAITH-BASED APPROACH: But how? The very first step is awareness. **Make a list containing all the foods that you have a tendency to indulge in.** It's important that you acknowledge their existence and the initial power that they have over you in order for you to break free from them.

Once you have your list ready, make sure that you're limiting the amount that you're consuming while making healthier options highly available. **Salt, added sugar, and trans fats** (cakes, margarine, chocolates, cookies, burgers, French fries, pastries, pizza, etc.), are options that are frequently mentioned as "addictive." Thus, instead of having these options available at all times, replace them with a variety of nuts and seeds, fruits and vegetables, coconut water, and natural ingredients.

NOTES

_____

_____

_____

_____

_____

_____

_____

_____

_____

_____

_____

_____

_____

_____

_____

_____

DAY 14

*"That each of them may eat and drink, and find
satisfaction in all their toil—this is the gift of God."*
Ecclesiastes 3:13 ESV

This verse is all about satisfaction, and so I'd like the opportunity to talk about fulfilling foods and empty calories. Most fast food or frozen food options that are easy and accessible are high in calories but lack nutritional content. Essentially, this means that you can eat a massive portion of them and not feel full.

You probably can relate to the feeling of eating a portion of French fries or a huge slice of cake but still wanting to keep eating. It's not because these food items are not providing you with the necessary calories, but that these calories are empty, and they do not provide the nutrients your body actually needs: **vitamins**. On the other hand, when you eat healthy meals, you feel instantly satisfied.

God wants us to feel gratitude for the food He has blessed us with, and that doesn't necessarily mean you can't eat your favorite cake once in a while. Instead, this scripture is a reminder to find joy in eating, and most importantly, find satisfaction.

FAITH-BASED APPROACH: When choosing the best foods to eat, one of the easiest options is to make sure that **you're consuming enough fiber**. Fiber isn't digested in your stomach. Instead, it passes through and ends up in your colon, where it essentially becomes food for beneficial gut bacteria.

By creating the perfect environment for good bacteria to grow, you promote a healthy gut, leading to weight loss, lower levels of blood sugar, and improved digestion. Here are some sources of fiber you can add to your meals:

- Avocado, Apples, Strawberries, Pears, Raspberries, Bananas, etc.
- Carrots, Beets, Broccoli, Artichoke, Brussels Sprouts, Lentils, Kidney Beans, etc.

NOTES

DAY 15

"No temptation has overtaken you that is not common to man. God is faithful, and he will not let you be tempted beyond your ability, but with the temptation, he will also provide the way of escape, that you may be able to endure it."
1 Corinthians 10:13 ESV

This is my absolute favorite verse about temptation because many of us can probably relate to the feeling of it in many different areas of our lives. It's tricky; that overwhelming sensation that we must surrender to our cravings immediately. When it comes to food, the strong feeling comes with a sense of urgency.

However, this urgency doesn't really exist. You're going to be fine! You don't really need to eat this ice cream so desperately, and it definitely will be fine if you don't devour this cheeseburger in five minutes. God is much more powerful than any temptation we might face, and we can always run to Him when in need of help. God doesn't promise us a life free of temptation, but He promises to show us a way out when we see Him.

This verse is important to remind us that God is faithful and that "giving in" to what seems to be irresistible temptation isn't the only option. You can always turn to God and ask for His guidance in moments of trouble.

FAITH-BASED APPROACH: When trying to avoid temptation in your diet, one of the best things you can do is focus on **Volume Eating** rather than calories. Volume eating is always about eating larger amounts of healthy food items that provide your body with the nutrients and vitamins it needs.

Volume eating is powerful because it eliminates the pressure of eating an abnormally small portion of food while still providing good weight loss results. Here is a small list of foods you can eat without worrying about the portion:

- Leafy Greens, Cruciferous Vegetables.
- Stem & Other Vegetables, Fruits;
- Root Vegetables, Whole Grains, Lean Cuts of Meat.

NOTES

_____

_____

_____

_____

_____

_____

_____

_____

_____

_____

_____

_____

_____

_____

_____

_____

_____

DAY 16

"But the fruit of the Spirit is love, joy, peace, patience,
kindness, goodness, faithfulness, gentleness, self-control;
against such things there is no law."
Galatians 5:22-23 ESV

For many people on weight loss journeys or simply trying to live a healthier lifestyle, it all comes down to discipline and self-control. This is why this verse is so important! It's crucial that, when trying to change our habits, we no longer lie to ourselves. We must instead recognize our eating behaviors, the efforts that are necessary for us to maintain these habits, and how they make us feel.

Often, people with binging issues, for example, can hide food from their loved ones, travel or commute long distances to buy a specific food that they are craving, and even take money in secret to maintain the addiction. All of those are issues with self-control. The characteristics listed in this verse are then crucial for our change to come from within.

This verse inspires me, and hopefully, you, to be kinder and happier, nurture our patience and goodness, but also practice self-control and discipline, even when it is hard. Of course, everyone has unique limitations, but everything is possible with God.

FAITH-BASED APPROACH: When speaking about the importance of discipline while also recognizing the unique limitations we all have, I find it particularly inspiring to discuss the possibility of doing everything at home. **At-home workouts can be just as effective** as the ones done at the gym because what matters the most is your determination and discipline. Exercise is exercise, no matter where you practice it.

NOTES

_____

_____

_____

_____

_____

_____

_____

_____

_____

_____

_____

_____

_____

_____

_____

_____

_____

DAY 17

"Jesus said to them, "I am the bread of life; whoever comes to me shall not hunger, and whoever believes in me shall never thirst."
John 6:35 ESV

Have you ever felt true hunger? That type of insatiable hunger that doesn't seem to go away no matter what you eat or what you do. The type of hunger that sneaks up on us after a busy day, when we are tired and thrown in our comfy beds and all we can think about is having tons of fast food? If so, are you sure this is actual physical hunger?

God would never leave us hungry, and those who seek Him will never be thirsty. But sometimes, it's easier to confuse spiritual hunger with physical hunger. Chances are, after a long day at work or taking care of the house, listening to so much noise, and taking care of everything that needs your attention, your body and heart are empty and in desperate need of a recharge. The type of energy that can't be provided with food.

This verse is a reminder to seek God in moments when you feel physically and spiritually empty and drained because He is the only one capable of satisfying your cravings and filling that void. It's also important to learn to recognize where your true hunger is coming from.

FAITH-BASED APPROACH: One of the main reasons why people overeat is their inability to recognize **real hunger cues**. We confuse frustration, tiredness, and that feeling of laziness with hunger when in reality, our body and Spirit can be craving God's word and presence. With this in mind, I've selected a short list of hunger cues that can help you identify if food is what you need:

- Stomach growling & the feeling of an empty stomach;
- Low energy & lack of focus;
- Shakiness & gradual increase of hunger cues;
- Headaches & irritability.

NOTES

_____

_____

_____

_____

_____

_____

_____

_____

_____

_____

_____

_____

_____

_____

_____

_____

_____

_____

DAY 18

"But don't be so concerned about perishable things like food. Spend
your energy seeking the eternal life that the Son of Man can give you.
For God, the Father has given me the seal of his approval."
John 6:27 NLT

In this passage, Jesus is warning those who had followed after Him in
search of his provisions instead of His person. He warns these people
that they shouldn't be blinded by the desire to get or have something,
but rather to seek Him and focus on creating a connection with Him in
His essence and not what He can offer.

Many people struggle with this. I have too! When we're spending hours
and hours worrying about what we're going to eat and what we're going
to do to exercise more… It's so easy to lose track of the things that really
matter. This obsessive behavior towards food can be a sign of an
unhealthy relationship with what you eat.

Do you feel guilty about what you're eating? Do you restrict yourself?
Do you use calorie-counting apps obsessively? Do you ignore your
body's hunger cues? Are you suffering from the yo-yo effect? All of these
signs can show that you have become obsessive with food and lost track
of what should've been the utmost priority: seeking God and the eternal
that only He can offer.

FAITH-BASED APPROACH: In order to start breaking these habits and change your relationship with food, we must start by changing the way you perceive food as a whole. There are no such things as "bad" or "good" foods, and no food should be off-limits. **Give yourself unconditional permission to eat** according to your hunger cues.

When you create a bunch of rules around food, you increase the risk of becoming obsessive and spending all of your energy deciding what you're going to eat or not. Following Mindful Eating practices, planning your meals ahead – so you don't have to think about food every day – and managing your pantry well are all helpful tips. **Maintainability** should be a priority!

NOTES

_____

_____

_____

_____

_____

_____

_____

_____

_____

_____

_____

_____

_____

_____

_____

_____

_____

DAY 19

"But I discipline my body and keep it under control, lest after preaching to others I myself should be disqualified."
1 Corinthians 9:27 ESV

You're reading this devotional because you want to be healthier and make your body stronger, and you understand that your choices should honor God. But this verse makes me think of how having a healthy body and mind is beneficial, not only on a personal level, but also because it is of great value to the Kingdom of God.

When we are well and healthy, we are able to produce good things. The opposite is also true. When we treat our bodies as if they are trash cans, then only trash enters and leaves our bodies. In this verse, Paul was aware that all of his efforts to become more disciplined meant that he was becoming qualified and stronger in order to live out God's calling.

Thus, whenever you're feeling discouraged and tempted to give up on this journey, think about this verse and what it truly means to see your body as God's Temple. Then, consider how you can honor Him by cherishing and nurturing the one and only body that was given to you so that you can open up and receive God's calling in your life.

FAITH-BASED APPROACH: As much as I tell you that it is possible to work out from home or go on daily walks, as suggested on days 11 and 16, I cannot simply close my eyes to the difficulty that some women might face while trying to squeeze in more activities in their daily lives. Thus, this is something that you can do every morning and that doesn't take more than a few minutes.

Personally, I believe in the benefits of **stretching and how powerful it can be for our bodies**. Low-impact practices such as Yoga and Pilates can often be done at home. However, if you can't even take 30 minutes to do an online class, stretching every day as soon as you wake up can already be a start!

NOTES

_____

_____

_____

_____

_____

_____

_____

_____

_____

_____

_____

_____

_____

_____

_____

_____

_____

_____

DAY 20

*"Because we have these promises, dear friends, let us cleanse
ourselves from everything that can defile our body or Spirit. And
let us work toward complete holiness because we fear God."*
2 Corinthians 7:1 NLT

While reading this verse and analyzing it, I invite you to think about the things that can defile your body and Spirit. Just like you might imagine, so many behaviors and habits can be harmful to both our spiritual and physical health, and it's crucial that we're mindful of them.

When it comes to our eating habits, eating large amounts of food, and foods that we know are damaging to our health is one of the easiest and most common examples of developing a behavior that can defile our bodies, putting our health at risk.

I know it's difficult, but start seeing food and your approach in regards to it as a behavior. When deciding what to eat, think not only about your physical health but also about your spiritual well-being. Avoid behaviors that you would be ashamed of exhibiting in front of others, and instead choose to live a proudful life in front of God. Thus, rid your life of the habits and foods that can put your happiness at stake.

FAITH-BASED APPROACH: When mentioning habits that can be damaging to our bodies and health, it's impossible not to mention sedentarism, which is why I want to introduce you to the concept of **NEAT - Non-exercise activity thermogenesis**. Essentially, this means expending more energy on your daily activities without actually exercising. This can be the biggest "trick" for busy women, as you can use it to burn more calories and energy while doing your day-to-day activities. I've selected a few suggestions:

- Housework! Yes, sweeping the house, mopping, washing dishes. You need energy for all of them. Declutter your closets, and move furniture around. Just make sure you're moving. Play outside with the kids, leave your phone far from you so that you can walk to it, stand more, walk your groceries home and so on.

NOTES

DAY 21

"When you sit down to eat with a ruler, observe carefully what is before you, and put a knife to your throat if you are given to appetite."
Proverbs 23:1-2 ESV

At first, this verse might sound a bit scary, but I challenge you to take a deeper look into what it means. Essentially, the message here is that we should be mindful of our appetites and keep it in check, not letting our cravings or desires control our lives and our actions. Although difficult, this verse encourages us to try to recover our self-control.

"I have self-control," you might think. But how often do you find yourself eating too much at lunch or dinner to the point where you feel bloated and experience the infamous "food coma"? How often do you let yourself go and eat that dessert even though you complained about being way too full just a couple of minutes before?

You might feel tempted to let it slide, thinking it's not a big deal. But in a long-term setting, constantly overeating can lead to health complications and weight gain, and it also displays a problem with self-control. We need to be honest with ourselves and God, above all, and recognize how damaging some of our habits can be, as this is the only way to change them and ensure our spiritual and physical wellbeing.

FAITH-BASED APPROACH: On day 17, we saw how to listen to our hunger cues, which would allow us to spot the difference between emotional and physical hunger. And in the case that you're actually hungry for food, there are countless ingredients that have great satiation power. These food items are all packed with nutrients that can fuel your body and **suppress hunger in a healthy way**. Thus, I've selected a short list you can be mindful of:

- Protein – Proteins lower the hunger hormone levels and can make you feel full for much longer;
- As you saw on day 14, fiber is great for improving digestion and regulating appetite;

NOTES

_____

_____

_____

_____

_____

_____

_____

_____

_____

_____

_____

_____

_____

_____

_____

_____

DAY 22

"The eyes of all look to you, and you give
them their food in due season."
Psalm 145:15 ESV

What would happen to your relationship with food if you turned to God for provision? While most of us are lucky to have more than enough food, we should still direct our gaze upward while making dietary choices.

"Lord, what do you want me to do?"

This verse encourages us to seek God in what we eat and to see our meals and diet not as a burden but as a way to become closer to Him, honor Him, and appreciate Him. In moments of doubt or struggle, look up to Him and ask Him for help. Ask Him to guide and show you the best way to glorify Him and your food choices, and worship Him in your exercises.

Think of this message as an incentive to not see healthy eating or exercising as a punishment. It isn't! Rather, taking care of your body is a way to empower yourself to reach for foods that will best nurture the body, as well as seek movements that genuinely bring joy to you and glory to God.

FAITH-BASED APPROACH: While prayers are extremely personal and unique to each of us and our struggles, here is a suggestion of **a prayer focused on changing eating habits to best glorify God and honor His body**.

Heavenly Father, I'm humbly here to thank You for giving me everything I need to thrive and serve You in this earthly body. I offer my body and Spirit to Your work and ask for Your help in this wellness journey. You tell us to run with discipline and endurance, and I'm determined to keep trying. However, I cannot help but feel weakened and in need of your guidance. Please Lord, teach me how to care for my body better. Remind me to make the best decisions for my health. Help me create a support system for this goal. Above all, please Lord, use this journey to bring me closer to You. I pray in Your Son's Holy name. Amen!

NOTES

_____

_____

_____

_____

_____

_____

_____

_____

_____

_____

_____

_____

_____

_____

_____

_____

DAY 23

"You keep him in perfect peace whose mind is
stayed on you because he trusts in you."
Isaiah 26:3 ESV

How many of your dieting and exercising habits – or lack of, are a result of extreme stress and anxiety that pushes you into seeking comfort in the most caloric and convenient food and behavior? How would your eating habits and lifestyle change if you had complete peace? If you were not a victim of stress and anxiety, and if you could only focus on your wellness…

This verse is a powerful reminder that ultimate peace lies with God and His word, and that He can solve all of our worries, put our hearts at rest, and that it is with Him that we can encounter comfort, peace, and happiness. It is through His words that we can soothe our troubled minds and silence our loud thoughts. Therefore, it is Him that we should seek at all times, not food.

Issues such as stress and anxiety are amongst the most frequent causes of obesity. Not only do high levels of stress mess up your hormone regulation, it also causes mood variations that are often the cause of your late-night visits to the fridge and pantry. But this can change!

FAITH-BASED APPROACH: One of the most efficient ways to reduce stress and anxiety caused by the everyday chaos in our lives is to exercise. But no need to worry! I'm not talking about long trips to the gym here either. Almost any form of activity can increase your fitness level and therefore reduce your stress.

This happens because of the release of endorphins. Known as the "happy neurotransmitters," as the name suggests, they are responsible for your mood and that "feel good" or euphoric sensation. The release of endorphins is directly related to the activity, which can be **ANY** kind, including yoga, walking, swimming, weightlifting, dancing, gardening, climbing up the stairs, and so on. Thus, make an effort to become more active in order to boost your endorphin levels.

NOTES

DAY 24

"A person without self-control is like a
city with broken-down walls."
Proverbs 25:28 NLT

A life without self-control is a life without meaning. The ability to discipline oneself brings about life, peace, and success. We're always in so much trouble if we do not exercise self-control. Thus, meditating on self-control in Bible passages can effectively convict us so that we can confess our difficulties, agree with God, and find the strength to persevere!

However, it's not easy to develop self-control. Titus 2:11-13 also reads that: *"For the grace of God has appeared, bringing salvation for all people, training us to renounce ungodliness and worldly passions, and to live self-controlled, upright, and godly lives in the present age."* This verse makes me think about the real motivation for any change in my life: God.

If you've come here because you believe you "have to" gain better self-control, I'd want you to reconsider. Don't try to impose disciplinary behaviors; instead, seek God's love and let Him restore your heart. And, of course, there are also countless things you can do yourself to improve your chances of success. One must be mindful of doing their parts and let God guide the way.

FAITH-BASED APPROACH: One of the main problems with self-control is that people lose the willpower to stick with a new habit after a few days of trying to develop one. That initial motivation to change their health fades away, and it is difficult to move forward. With this in mind, I have listed a few tips that can increase the chances of success in your new wellness journey:

- Finding ways to burn more calories by doing the things you already do is much simpler than finding a new activity.
- Make exercising as easy as possible. Avoid classes that are far away. Instead, make the process as convenient as possible. You can also prepare your outfit, snacks, and everything you'll need for your morning workout session the night before!

NOTES

_____

_____

_____

_____

_____

_____

_____

_____

_____

_____

_____

_____

_____

_____

_____

_____

_____

DAY 25

"There is nothing outside a person that by going into him can defile him, but the things that come out of a person are what defile him." Do you not see that whatever goes into a person from outside cannot defile him, since it enters not his heart but his stomach, and is expelled."
Mark 7:15, 18-19 ESV

Lastly, I wanted to invite you to look at your own behavior with regards to food. Do you ever feel like you just committed a crime because you ate something that you thought you shouldn't? Did you ever feel the need to punish yourself because you weren't able to follow a diet plan that you had set for yourself? Do you consider food your worst enemy?

I love this verse because there are so many of us who are struggling with this never-ending cycle. You start to follow a very restrictive diet, you manage to stick to it for a few days, and then you make a "mistake." You feel horrible. You think of yourself as less. You think you committed the worst of crimes because you ate something that was "bad."

However, this verse reminds us that there is no such thing. To God, you are NOT what you eat. It is simply not how He works. The most important thing, at the end of the day, is your heart and your God-glorifying actions. God is merciful, a source of strength, and He will always be the one to forgive us our sins. Thus, always remember to be kind to yourself.

FAITH-BASED APPROACH: Throughout this devotional, you've seen so many Mindful Eating tips and tricks, as well as information that can be used to develop a healthier relationship. For our last day, **I've written a prayer about healthy eating, weight loss, and food addiction.** Read it carefully:

Dear Heavenly God, I've struggled with my weight and overeating for a long time. Today, I finally confess that I have no control over my overeating and food addiction. When I'm anxious, fatigued, bored, overwhelmed, or lonely, I overeat. My eating is indeed uncontrollable and out of control. I now understand what it means to be "powerless." Please God, help me quit my food addiction and allow me to heal. I ask for Your help and guidance. Amen!

KEEP GOING:
IT'S A JOURNEY

I t is very common, in a Christian environment, to see people take very good care of their spiritual life and even of their souls. They do it because they understand that there is a divine order in this sense. However, some can neglect the care of the body, focusing only on the spiritual aspect, as it is deemed eternal. On the other hand, the body is a temporary vessel, which leads many people to believe it doesn't deserve as much care and attention. However, this highlights a certain ignorance regarding the biblical truths that guide this subject, which is what ultimately motivated me to write **Health Beyond Lip Service.**

The word of God reveals to us that we have three parts: **Body, Soul, and Spirit**. This truth is expressed clearly and unquestionably in 1 Thessalonians 5:23 ESV: *"Now may the God of peace himself sanctify you completely, and may your whole spirit and soul and body be kept blameless at the coming of our Lord Jesus Christ."* Thus, when trying to understand the importance of taking care of our body, one cannot simply leave aside this incredible revelation left by the Holy Spirit.

Although it is true that our main concern is to do God's will, one must recognize that taking care of our bodies is also His wish. Recalling 1 Thessalonians 5:23: *"Now may the God of peace himself sanctify you completely, and may your whole spirit and soul and body be kept blameless at the coming of our Lord Jesus Christ."* The word of God affirms that our three bodies must be kept intact and blameless until Christ returns. So everything is important!

> *But if God made us in three bodies and only two of them are eternal, why also take care of what is our temporary abode? Should we pay equal attention to the three bodies?*

Doubts like these need to be addressed; as we saw in each of our **25-Days devotional journeys**, there are so many biblical passages about caring for God's temple. Our greatest example is Jesus, who was certainly an athlete and ate very well, as he would not be able to complete his ministry in a city or walk after filling his belly with "McDonald's" or "In & Out." He walked many kilometers a day moving to where the Spirit impelled Him, and in the same way, His disciples who walked with Him and the crowd that followed Him in search of miracles. Thus, we can safely conclude that the people of that time **were not sedentary**.

Nowadays, what we can sometimes observe in the Christian environment is the total paralysis of the body's functions in the context of poor diet and habits, which results in a lot of fatigue, laziness, and diseases affecting the people of God. But yet again, the answer can be found in God's word. Let's see what the apostle Paul tells us about this:

As mentioned on the very first day of our devotional: "1 Corinthians 6:19-20, *"Or do you not know that your body is a temple of the Holy Spirit within you, whom you have from God? You are not your own, for you were bought with a price. So glorify God in your body."* This is an exhortation of God coming through Paul to the church of Corinth where he essentially says: "Do you not know...", bringing to the memory of those people something already known or easily assimilated, **that their body was not their own**, but a **sanctuary of God**, and should be cared for and exposed in such a way that it glorifies its owner, Him.

And as we've seen, body care ranges from external to internal factors. That is, changing our diets, nurturing a healthier relationship with food, practicing self-control and discipline, eating foods from the earth, and giving thanks to Him for the food provided.

Thus, we need to be concerned with how we present ourselves before the world, doing so in a way that is both balanced and free from vanity or the desire to "force" a particular status, because the word teaches us: 1 Corinthians 6:12 ESV *"All things are lawful unto me, but all things are not expedient: all things are lawful for me, but I will not be brought under the power of any."*

Also, 1 Timothy 4:8 informs us that: *"For bodily exercise profiteth little: but godliness is profitable unto all things, having promise of the life that now is, and of that which is to come."* Note that this verse does not say that exercise is worthless, rather it says that exercise has some value, while the ultimate priorities lie in godliness, which carries the greater value.

Ultimately, the Bible makes it clear that we should **take good care of our bodies** (1 Corinthians 6:19-20 ESV). Ephesians 5:29 NLT tells us, *"No one hates his own body but feeds and cares for it, just as Christ cares for the church. And we are members of his body."* The Bible also warns us against **gluttony** (Deuteronomy 21:20; Proverbs 23:2; 2 Peter 1:5-7; 2 Timothy 3:1-9; 2 Corinthians 10: 5). At the same time, the Bible warns us against **vanity** (1 Samuel 16:7; Proverbs 31:30; 1 Peter 3:3-4).

Thus, **be healthy**! And I hope that the daily inspiration provided in this devotional helped you get closer to God as you took care of His temple and helped you develop a healthier relationship with His biggest gift. Feel welcome to use this devotional to kick start a long-lasting healthy and wellness journey alongside His word. I sincerely hope you are able to follow the biblical standard for health and exercise.

www.ingramcontent.com/pod-product-compliance
Lightning Source LLC
Chambersburg PA
CBHW052025030426
42335CB00026B/3284